Aurea Vidyā Collection*

–––––––– 3 ––––––––

*For a complete list of Titles, see page 60

BEYOND THE ILLUSION OF THE EGO

This book was originally published in Italian
as *Oltre l'illusione dell'io*
by Edizioni Āśram Vidyā, Roma

First published in English in 2001 by
Aurea Vidyā
39 West 88th Street, New York, N.Y. 10024, U.S.A.
www.vidya-ashramvidyaorder.org

© Āśram Vidyā 1995
  Second Edition 1996
  English translation © Āśram Vidyā 2001

Set in font ©Vidyā 12/12 points by Edizioni Āśram Vidyā

Printed and bound by Lighntning Source Inc. at locations in the
U.S.A and in the U.K. as shown on the last page.

ISBN 10: 1-931406-03-0

ISBN 13: 978-1-931406-03-1

Library of Congress Control Number: 2001098284

RAPHAEL

(Āśram Vidyā Order)

BEYOND THE ILLUSION
OF THE EGO

Synthesis of a Realizative Process

AUREA VIDYĀ

«Reality is not outside of Being, but within Being. The efforts are, therefore, aimed at conquering the truth of the Self, the essential nature of the supreme Reality»

Raphael

TABLE OF CONTENTS

FOREWORD

In the introduction to *The Threefold Pathway of Fire* [1] we read: «Raphael's "Pathway of Fire" is the operative way that leads to the lighting of the Fire, to the mastery and direction of the Fire, and then to the extinction of that same Fire».

As this small book intends to offer only a synthetic approach of the process leading to realization, whoever wishes to gain a deeper knowledge of this matter should refer to the book mentioned above, where three operational paths are prospected:

a) Realization according to Alchemy (Section I, Chapter 1)

b) Realization according to Love of Beauty (Section I, Chapter 2)

c) Realization according to Traditional Metaphysics (Section I, Chapter 3)

When an aspirant is stimulated to undertake the Way leading to the realization of the Self, when he or she is no longer interested in the multitude of books available on the most varied subjects and has ceased talking haphazardly of spiritual things, his consciousness demands of him a more

---

[1] Raphael, *The Threefold Pathway of Fire*, Aurea Vidyā, New York.

operative and decisive action, aimed at solving his restless yearnings. At this point, from a vague wandering, a searching here and there, he will move on to the concrete application of his *sādhanā* (realizative ascesis) and to the choice of a Path that is most congenial to his psychological state.

What is suggested in this small book is an *operational synthesis* that may be taken as the basic scheme for any possible *sādhanā*.

For one who is ready, this operational synthesis could prove to be sufficient to raise him to the realization of that Being that *is* and does not become. For one who is mature, just a few indications are sufficient to enable him to put his wings back on and fly to Freedom.

If an ens[1] (integral being) lives in conflict, in material and psychological suffering, restlessness and dissatisfaction, it means that something is not working within himself, or something is wrong in his life conduct. It may be that his way of living rests on an incorrect vision of existence, that he is following a dead-end philosophy of life, so much that he resigns himself and proceeds by force of inertia, or passively conforms to the chaotic collective unconscious, without any prospect of ever emerging from it.

Yet, without a doubt, there are optimal solutions for the restless and anguished human being. But one should be more responsive, more flexible, more humble and ready to listen to a voice which one is unlikely to run into in this world of dichotomy.

But what is a realizative Way, if not one that unveils the Fullness and Knowledge of oneself? These things can be

---

[1] Refer to Glossary

found within the ens himself but they stay deeply hidden within the hollow of one's heart, the attention often being focused more on the world of becoming than on the world of Being.

What can we give to others, if our own life is interwoven with emotions, passions, and egotism, and if we ignore the various existential problems? Often we cannot even give psychological comfort to help them carry on.

Maturity, that is often gained under the hammer of suffering, sooner or later will force us to remove the Eye of intelligence from things that *are not* (world of duality) and direct it toward the splendor of one's own essential nature. Undoubtedly, this implies an overturning of values, a psychological revolution, tending no longer toward the ineffective and unfruitful horizontal line, but toward the vertical one leading to awakening, to the unveiling of marvelous potentialities, which are the prerogative of the human soul.

This operational synthesis is dedicated to those who, having matured under the law of *necessity*, now want to taste the admirable path of Freedom, until they themselves *are* Freedom-completeness. It is only then that we can offer to others not simple psychological comfort, but something more.

The Fire that we have mentioned is naturally not the one we know on the physical level. Instincts, passions, ideas, etc., are nothing but expressions of fire: our bodies in manifestation (physical, emotional and mental) are made up of fire, and also matter is a concentrate of fire. A star is fire that sheds light; life itself can be understood in terms of fire. *Yoga* speaks of seven centers of consciousness that express energy-fire-light. Some of these have to be awakened so that the energy-fire may rise along a specific line and lead the consciousness to the universal dimension.

The life of a disciple is, therefore, a life of fire. At the beginning this can be disturbing, so much so that he may even refuse this fire that seems unknown to him, since he has never considered himself in terms of fire.

But when the disciple awakens, the fire imposes itself on him, and he is forced to acknowledge it. This might be difficult at the outset, because he does not know how to handle this element, nor how to face up to it.

This happens only because *avidyā* (non-knowledge of one's own essential nature) hides from us the fundamental fact that, from the field of tension that proceeds from the universal Principle to the heart of formal matter, everything is fire.

When the disciple gradually discovers his own reality of Fire, he is freed thanks to that fire. He recognizes himself as Fire and by constantly burning on the stake he eliminates whatever emerges between him and his essence. Thus he learns to reject all that cannot be sustained in the breath of fire.

May this short treatise be of help to all of those who are approaching the realization of the Self.

Aurea Vidyā

BEYOND THE ILLUSION OF THE EGO

«I will give you the keys to open the doors of the Temple. In It you will find the regenerating Fire that will make you expand as much as creation, the flaming sword to fight the binding darkness and the resplendent and constant Truth»

Raphael

INTRODUCTION

The three individuated fires[1] are powerful qualified energies of an "ego" in relation with another "ego". One can be polarised on a specific energetic quality, primarily. We therefore have individuals that are strictly instinctual, emotional-sentimental-passional, or mental. Or we could also have an ego with mixed qualities. But it is important to remember that at this level the fires are always related to an ego center. As long as the reflection of consciousness of the pure Self-*Noûs* identifies with such fires it cannot be free to go back to the Source. To say it with Plotinus, this reflection moved away from the Source owing to simple "temerity", i.e. due to its freedom to move in multiple directions.

Therefore, the whole process leading to realization consists in appropriate operational phases:

1. Comprehension of the individuated fires.

2. Separation of the reflection of soul consciousness (*jīva*) from its own projections.

3. Fixing of the Center of consciousness upon itself.

---

[1] Refer to the symbol on page 21

4. Overturning of the Center of consciousness, and therefore integration of the individuated fires, toward the universal and principial counterpart of the fires.

5. Capturing of the Essence of Fire and stabilizing of the Awareness on such metaphysical state.

In synthesis, the *reflection of consciousness* – individuated and separated from the context of Being, and thus identified with the world of simple appearances – regains its authentic universal nature. The parable of the Prodigal Son returning home is emblematic.

The human ens is a luminous spiritual center, but, because of his own free will to act, he may lose his splendor. He can step down into the "cave" and see nothing but the shadow of Reality – even though this is a relative event, since the being, obviously, cannot change its nature.

The immortal cannot become mortal but may nevertheless "think" himself and "believe" himself to be finite and corruptible. For example, by identifying with the contingent gross-physical body, the immortal Soul may consider itself mortal, but this event can be only apparent and non-real.

Essence of Fire

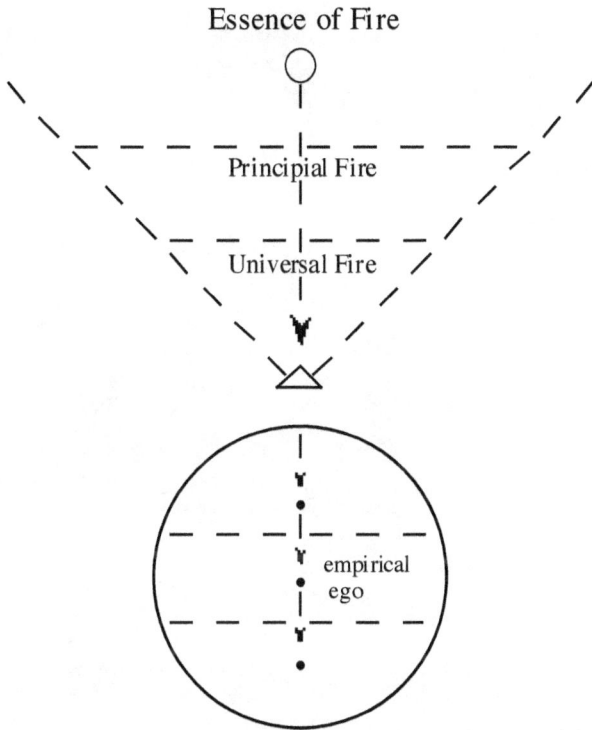

Principial Fire

Universal Fire

empirical
ego

AWAKENING

TO THE REALIZATION OF THE SELF

1. The Fire we are talking about bears no reference to the fire element proper. It has a much deeper meaning: It is the very essence of manifestation and it permeates our formal nature. We have to light it, dominate it, direct it, so that the obstructing accumulations may be totally burnt.

Alchemy, but Yoga as well, speak of Fire.

In *The Pathway of Fire according to the Qabbālāh*, we read: «To extinguish the threefold Fire one needs to have maturity, dignity, ardor and intuitive knowledge.

He who has extinguished the threefold Fire, and has a body still, is a "living corpse" (liberated in life).

A "living corpse" leaves no signs or footsteps, has no *goal* to attain, nor profane *duty* to fulfil.

He who is Complete lives only of Completeness and of Fullness, and this Fullness is unconnected with any determination, action or aim»[1].

---

[1] Raphael, *La via del Fuoco secondo la Qabbālāh*, Edizioni Āśram Vidyā, Roma. Published in English as: Raphael, *The Pathway of Fire* - Initiation to the Kabbalah, S. Weiser, York Beach, Me. U.S.A.

2. «"Oh Yama, you who know of the Fire that leads to Heaven, reveal it to me, who am full of faith".

"I will teach you that Fire, oh Naciketas, that can raise you up to Heaven. Know that Fire is the means by which to attain infinite worlds; It is their very foundation and It is hidden in a secret place".

He then revealed to him that Fire, source of the world ».

(*Kaṭha Upaniṣad*: I, 13-15)

The disciple to the Pathway of Fire must have specific qualifications. Without them he may fall prey to misunderstandings and illusion. Therefore it is necessary:

a) To work on the transformation of one's own Temple, because it has been rendered no longer sacred.

b) To be reserved in an intelligent and measured way: the opus must not be disturbed by external factors. This implies avoiding the dispersion of the Fires, but instead concentrating them fully on the opus of transformation. Therefore, think and speak only when need requires, and act only when duty is mandatory.

c) To operate no matter what Life's social and profane circumstances may be. The Opus does not allow for extenuating circumstances nor for delays.

d) To understand that every individual expresses *qualities*, or energies of various kind and color, which means that in time-space everything is in its right place. This implies non-contraposition.

e) To ask oneself right questions, whilst bearing in mind that many questions have no answer. Some others are badly put, other still are asked prematurely. A correct position of consciousness predisposes to the right kind of questions. A true dialogue with oneself, or with an Instructor, can only take place when questions are asked in the right way.

f) To work not for a reward. If there is any request for a reward, then one should know that the ego's hand is behind the request, that very ego which one should instead either "incinerate" or integrate.

g) To remember that the way to immortality is not made of doubts, of postponement, of self-commiseration and of fears. The "Pathway of Fire" is for those who know how to dare and to drop all prejudice.

3. All of this implies that the Pathway of Fire is operational, positive and realizative. Without lighting the Fire within one's own Temple, one cannot proceed. It is good to recognize this from the very beginning in order to avoid all future disappointments.

If some qualifications are still not there, they may be encouraged through the *technique of evocation*. All is already in us, but some things are at the potential level, and they have to be called to actuality.

4. The world of *avidyā*, or the condensed fire, does not lead to solutions. It has no finality, and it disappears at the moment of the *Awakening*.

5. The incarnate reflection of consciousness, according to the *Vedānta* Tradition, has five sheaths or bodies-vases that operate on three universal levels of life: the gross, the subtle and the causal level. The sheaths-bodies are different

condensations of Fire, but the unawakened human being considers himself as being just the physical sheath. From the metaphysical perspective, the three states and the five sheaths are nothing but *appearance* in that they appear on the formal horizon and then disappear.

6. Fire can operate on three dimensions. It can be at the purely gross-physical, material or condensed level, at the fluid or subtle radiant level, and at the noumenic level.

Consequently, a living Soul may experience three states of consciousness which find their expression on three levels of Fire.

When, for example, a Soul leaves its gross physical body, it finds itself clothed in the subtle and the noumenic bodies. When it leaves the subtle body (second death) it will find itself only with the focal noumenic principle. When this one dissolves, by means of metaphysical Knowledge, the Consciousness rests in its non-qualified nature.

7. Pure Consciousness is all-pervading, therefore it is immanent and at the same time transcendent. It is within and without. It is above and below.

This is the reason why the individuated reflection of consciousness must resolve into unlimited all-pervasiveness, or, in other words, it must rejoin that Source with which in reality it never parted.

Liberation, therefore, is bursting out of chains, of limitations, of restraints, of necessity and of identification. If the being's essence rests on freedom of choice, then one among the indefinite number of choices may be that of finding oneself in a specific condition, even if it implies conflicting duality.

8. On the other hand, the individual's antinomy is brought about by a "dissatisfaction of being", by a restlessness that drives him to search along paths that are further prisons. The satisfaction of emotions, volitions and appetites is the effect of the scissure from his divine counterpart. It is the portion, as reflection, that is in search of its totality. Therefore, man's restlessness is legitimate. What is wrong is the direction of his search.

This is represented by the myth of Narcissus who, by looking at his mirrored image, identifies himself with his "shadow", and by "losing himself" in the shadow, forgets the Source.

Incarnate awareness, through the mental vehicle, appears "other" than itself. The mind acts as *māyā*, as the mirror, just as the water for Narcissus represents the substance that causes his reflection to appear. Identification with this reflection causes his "fall". So, the mental substance is the *medium* in which the *Puruṣa*'s reflection appears.

Plato's Tradition, and therefore the Mysteries', rightly speaks of *remembrance*, i.e. calling back into our own memory our real identity. The dream state is a significant analogy for understanding the mechanism of projection and of identification (*vikṣepa śakti* and *āvaraṇa śakti*).

9. The problem of human suffering is one of *scissure* which brings about duality, which in turn is the source of conflict, of ego and non-ego, of attraction-repulsion and so on.

Closing the scissure means recomposing oneself into oneness, being a one all and regaining one's own integrity.

10. Realization is, therefore, *awakening* to what one is from eternity. It is to become aware of the noumenic Fire and then of the non-qualified one as the absolutely *constant* polar Point. As a consequence, it is not by proceeding along horizontal lines of impermanent becoming and movement that we may find ourselves, but it is on the vertical plane. It is not by *going* that we will find Freedom but by *stopping*.

11. Therefore, our fundamental problem is to *awaken*. Rather than looking for some "ideology" to save the world, we should comprehend what we are, what our true immortal Essence is. The rest will obviously follow.

If one is not inflamed with the sacred fire of Being it is not possible to follow the "Pathway of Fire". We cannot fly if we do not spread our wings. We cannot irradiate if we do not light our Fire.

12. From the point of view of the absolute Knowledge (*paravidyā*) there is but one Reality: the non-qualified and non-determined Fire. From the point of view of sensorial or empirical knowledge (*aparavidyā*) there is a prime Cause, and many effects.

The realization of the being develops along an *experimental* line that goes from the awareness of multiplicity to the awareness of the One-principle and on to the unveiling of Reality without a second.

To say it with Plato, we move from the One *and* the many (sensible world) to the One-many (world of Being) and finally to the One-One or One-Good, that is to say, the metaphysical non-qualified and non-determined One.

13. The analytical mind (*diánoia*) is the instrument that rectifies the qualities, while the superconscious mind (*nóesis*) is the instrument that unveils the universals and that integrates them into pure Consciousness.

14. On the "Pathway of Fire" we have to adapt our vision to that of the Truth-constant. But the dianoetic mind, under the impression of the ego, wants to adapt truth to its own partial and distorted vision. To be able to die to oneself what is needed is courage. Our "conception" of incompleteness is tenacious. Just when you think you have fought it off, it springs forth once again and blooms, as if our action had barely touched it.

15. On the other hand, speaking to you who are reading and who are ready, you cannot worry about what the others say. The world of the ego has to say something, but it no longer represents the food for your livelihood.

However, if you expect that the teaching is intended to satisfy unconscious requirements of the ego, then forget the Way, it is not yet for you.

16. It may be worth repeating that through the "Pathway of Fire" you will come, first of all, to master your focal Center, then to solve your condensed Fire, to experience the all-pervading Fire and finally, to resolve yourself into the non-qualified Fire, or into the very essence of the Fire.

The focal Center represents your directional pole, around which your psycho-physical fires rotate.

The individuated condensed Fire represents your "appearance".

The all-pervading Fire unveils for you the reality of Unity; the very essence of Fire unveils to you the one-without-a-second, because the second, whatever dimension or grade it may belong to, has been resolved and integrated into the One-One.

17. Comprehension of the psycho-physical fires, their coordination and integration, formation of a single Fire and then direction of the sole Fire; all of this is the essential motion of the "Pathway of Fire".

Below is a demonstrative table one needs to work on:

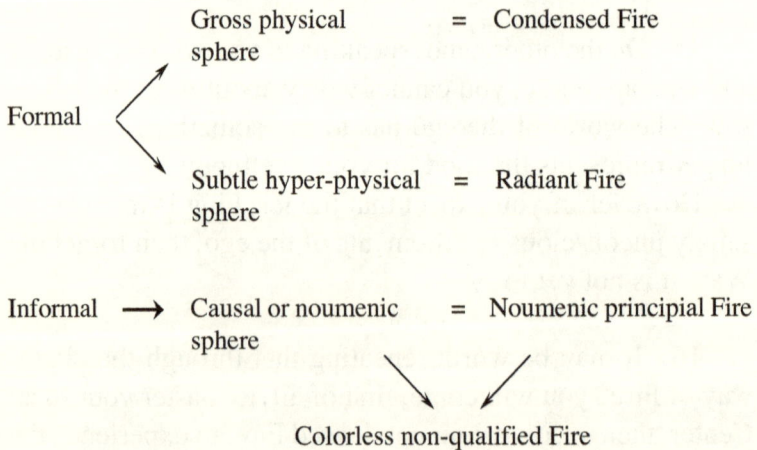

	Gross physical sphere	= Condensed Fire
Formal		
	Subtle hyper-physical sphere	= Radiant Fire
Informal ⟶	Causal or noumenic sphere	= Noumenic principial Fire
	Colorless non-qualified Fire	

At the microcosmic level we have:

Gross body   =   Fire of the physical dense state

Subtle body   =   Radiant Fire

State of pure Consciousness   =   Colorless non-qualified Fire

18. How can we, for example, dominate and then transcend the individuated thought? To comprehend this process it is helpful to understand first of all how the mind works. Let us imagine the mind as a vibrating substance-energy that, through its rhythm, can take different forms with indefinite qualitative features. Let us compare the mind with clay: with it we can mold different forms, such as vases, jars, statues and so on. Likewise the mental substance gives shape and rhythm to *images* which are then conceptualized or represented by means of ideas and concepts.

Let us stop on this word "image". In fact, when we think, we formulate images and rhythms which adhere to the various objects. So, when we observe a tree we mold our mind in the image of that tree. In other words, we adapt our substance to the rhythms of the tree.

We may even shut our eyes and see this image within our mind space (this process is called visualization). Our mental substance does nothing else but to "take the form" of the objects perceived and observed.

We said that the mind carries out another function: that of ideating and conceptualizing, i.e. it transforms the image or the object in terms of concept and then, in order to be able to communicate and transmit verbally, of language.

Also, in order to form the idea or the image of a tree, to capture the shape of the tree, to get hold of it and to mold itself accordingly, the mind has to emerge from itself. It has to leave its state of quiet.

Thus we have the following sequence:

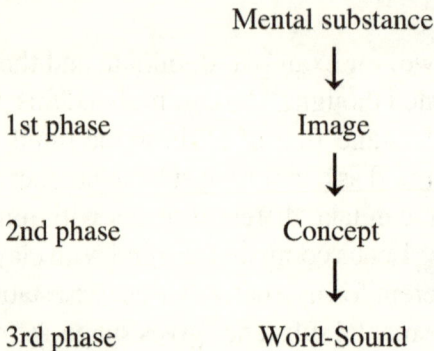

	Mental substance
	↓
1st phase	Image
	↓
2nd phase	Concept
	↓
3rd phase	Word-Sound

19. The mental image of the tree, of course, acts as the object and if there is an object, there must be a subject. These two are always interrelated and interdependent. Also, if we have a direct experience of the entire process, we will notice that this subject changes with the changing of events-things. The same subject can be joyful, sad, euphoric, etc. The subject that was sad is contradicted by the subject that is now happy, etc. An object can cause first happiness and then sadness in the same subject. Ego and non-ego are always relational data, they are moving and therefore aleatory. We can come to the conclusion that the subject and the object are psychological states, and therefore they are time-space. If

they are movements there must consequently be something that is stable, something which perceives and connects the different movements. This something is the consciousness, which is, precisely, conscious of the various alternating motions of the subject and the object.

So we have:

$$\text{Consciousness} \left\{ \begin{array}{l} \text{subject} \\ \\ \text{object} \end{array} \right.$$

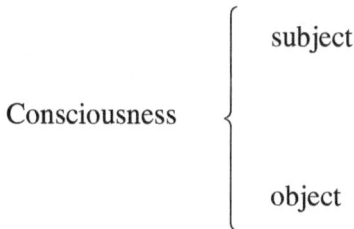

Thus, out of the three, because it is present during the different mental modifications, the consciousness emerges as the constant, even when the mind itself is quiet. In fact, we occasionally recognize that sometimes there are no thoughts, i.e. that we have not "projected" the subject and object. This is the state of pure consciousness, beyond time, space and cause.

20. So in what way can we dominate and transcend the relational and, therefore, individuated mind?

From what we have said, it can be deduced that the result can be obtained by "separating" the subject-object from the consciousness, and to then "fix" the very consciousness upon itself. In so doing consciousness-awareness becomes the absolute master of the dualistic movement to the point of stopping this movement, at will. It is at this point that you can recognize that out of the three the only reality-constant is the consciousness, which is ipseity. This is to say that it depends on none other but itself. The ego-world has disappeared. The two factors, becoming and relativity, are resolved, integrated, transcended.

21. It may happen that psychological contents appear within our inner space. More precisely, these contents are qualified energy coagulates possessing a certain amount of power and persistence sufficient to condition our center of consciousness, which is not yet stabilized. In fact, there are some particular contents-coagulates that may totally enslave and frustrate the ens. Each individual has his own "guardian of the threshold" to contend with, at times there may be more than one, and our consciousness might have great difficulty in trying to keep its balance.

What can we do in these cases? Let us put forward a few operative methods:

a) Through the power of sound (*mantra*), we can disaggregate the coagulate. This is an immediate, precise and dynamic act.

b) We can accept and integrate it into pure consciousness; of course, to enact this, we would need to have a suitable and solar state of consciousness.

c) We can slow down the rhythm of that content, and remove energy from it, and in so doing neutralize it completely.

d) We can use an energy possessing a quality which opposite to that of the coagulate. In this case we will obtain a sort of alchemic transmutation.

22. But what we have to avoid is to fight that content in a frontal way. The four methods of operation must be expressed with "determined calmness", with aware and loving firmness. It is not egoic will, but the *awareness* determined to arbitrate the event. In addition, we should not judge or blame, nor justify the content.

The Vision according to which all that which we perceive in our psychic space is nothing but a relative "second", albeit with a quite substantial consistency, is able to promote a more a solar type of consciousness. Only *one* who perceives, observes and is aware, who is *witness* to every qualitative movement, is Absolute; and when we become aware of our own absoluteness our attitude towards the "second" changes completely, and the solution of that event becomes certainty.

From this perspective we can say that traditional Knowledge is a fifth operative method. In fact, for those who are thus predisposed, Knowledge is sufficient to devitalize, neutralize and dissolve any possible "second" that may appear on the horizon of our psychic circumference. The *mantra* disintegrates the form, Knowledge belittles and dissolves, Love (that stems from the incarnate *puruṣa*) draws to itself all it touches, integrating and resolving all.

23. How does a psychological content, or an energy coagulate, take birth? To better understand this process, we may refer to the *Vedānta* vision, briefly focussing on the *puruṣa prakṛti* polarity. The *puruṣa* is the positive aspect, the Essence, while *prakṛti* is the substance, the energy (*chóra* in Platonic terms) out of which the different forms are shaped. *Māyā* is the substance through which forms appear to our perception.

As we have said, a psychological content is a qualified energy coagulate. This means that the incarnate *puruṣa* (the immanent Ray) through the *molding* mind, which is substance, shapes the content and qualifies it according to its own conscious or unconscious intention. Therefore, a qualified thought of whatsoever nature continually presented to the mind and repeated persistently creates, as a mater of fact, a *condensation* of the substance and finally forms an *entity*, as Plotinus calls it, able to condition the reflection of the *puruṣa*.

"We become what we think, this is the eternal mystery" says the *Maitry Upaniṣad*, or, in a more Western way, energy follows thought. Now we can understand the need to control our mind, so that it may become a docile instrument in the hands of the essential Ens.

24. We should remember that a realizative process consists in *dissolving* coagulated forms (qualitative individuated contents), slowing down the movement of *prakṛti*, and then resolving *prakṛti* into *puruṣa*. Substance is but a mere polarity. In this connection, the symbology of Adam and Eve is significant. Eve-substance is born out of the rib of Adam-essence. We can also say that the one, by projecting a reflection of his, creates the two; or again, the dot, by dividing, forms a line.

On the way of return, formal *quantity* (the multiplicity of contents of any order or degree) has to be reduced to unity, and the unity must be reintegrated in the One-without-a-second.

Conflict-pain derives from the contrast between the different psychological contents, as these have opposing qualities. It is quite evident that in our psychological space there are entities which we have created ourselves and which are fighting each other for their own survival.

We must quieten the many different voices that cloud and storm our consciousness. Without any sentimentalism, it is necessary to recognize that, it is either the substance that fills up all of our psychological circumference in a chaotic way, or the *puruṣa*, the real, essential ens, which imposes its rhythm and direction to our circumference.

Substance is a bad master, but it is an excellent and useful servant. To allow the *prakṛti* to be shaped by the diverse internal or external stimulations that it can receive, without a direction imparted by the essential Ens or "inner Orderer", is equivalent to being completely alienated.

The disorder in a society is the reflection-mirror of the disorder in the individual substance which is not shaped in accordance with pure Ideas, as Plato would say, or with the spiritual will of the Consciousness.

Ignorance of what one is (*avidyā*) leads to a life of psychotic projections, and therefore to 'insane' living. In fact, the world of empirical egos is a paranoid dimension. The Liberated has defeated ignorance. His life is without projections, without expectations: even his very actions may appear important in the eyes of others, but not in his own.

25. When you – and I am still speaking to you who are reading and are ready – have dissolved the different contents or indefinite qualified forms, you find in your circumference, on the one hand the incarnate *puruṣa*, and on the other hand, *prakṛti*, totally whole, neutral, non-qualified. If you are still thirsting for unity and completeness, you have to resolve (as you have already noticed) the *prakṛti* into *puruṣa*, so that the two become one.

At this point you can no longer say "I am this" ("this" refers to the many different contents and qualities that have characterised your psychic space). There is no second with whom you can identify. Since you have eliminated "this" you are just "I am". In fact you are simply "Am". You are at a very advanced state of consciousness because you have brought yourself to the primordial condition before the "fall" or before the "scissure", and you have solved even the "sense of ego" (*ahaṁkāra*) or the sense of belonging to a name and form.

This "Am" is the prime cause that can move in the multiple states of the universal Being in perfect freedom, and it can have indefinite possibilities of expression; it is the optimal state. But every cause is already in itself a determination. Although principle, which has originated all possible becoming, it represents the root of bondage, of the events that become concrete.

So we have:

Am   = Existence in manifestation as primordial cause

I am   = Awareness of the existence of a *me*

I am this = The *me* identified with the projections offered
                  by "I am"

26. The waking, dreaming and sleeping states, all of which are movement, are the states relevant to the "I am this", "I am" or "Am", respectively. The absolute awareness is the witness of the three states, and of the movement of existence and non-existence of the three states.

So the Being, in that it is and does not become, (absolute Consciousness) is not beyond just time and space, but also beyond the cause or the principle from which all emerges. So it is necessary to solve the "Am" (as the principle-universal consciousness, seed of the indefinite states of the ens) into the absolute, non-determined Reality.

We can say that the "Am" is the first determination, or specification, of the non-qualified Being-without-a-second, or metaphysical One.

Here we have a synopsis:

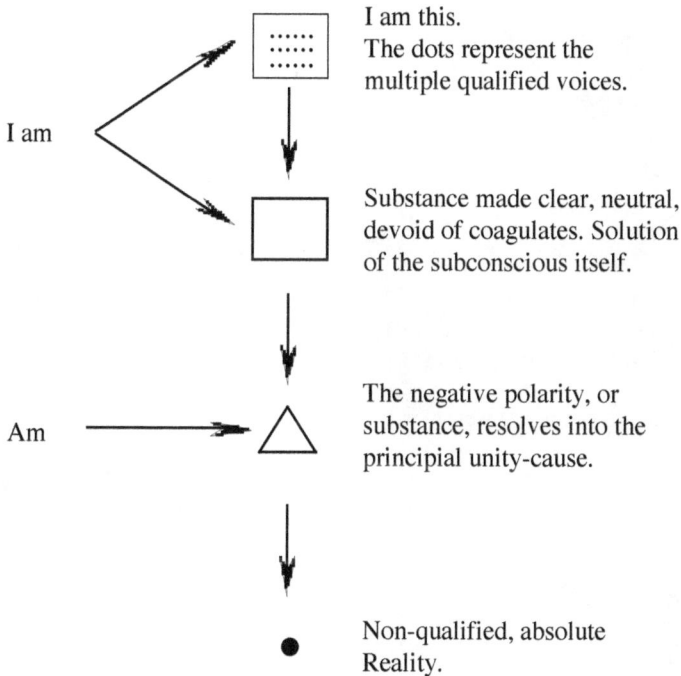

I am this.
The dots represent the
multiple qualified voices.

I am

Substance made clear, neutral,
devoid of coagulates. Solution
of the subconscious itself.

The negative polarity, or
substance, resolves into the
principial unity-cause.

Am

Non-qualified, absolute
Reality.

27. We could consider what has been said so far from another point of view. There is the all-pervading Ether (*Īśvara*-Being) which takes indefinite forms-sheaths (= One-many, according to Plato). That "part" of Ether which is inside a sheath-vase may identify with the different bodies-vehicles (gross-physical, mental, buddhic, etc.), thereby believing itself to be separate from both the universal Ether and the different ethers that are circumscribed in other sheaths-vases. Therefore it considers itself as "I am this" in opposition with the other entia (see glossary).

Realization consists in no longer identifying with the different bodies-sheaths-vases, and all of their specific qualities, to the point of recognizing oneself as "I am Ether" (and no longer body-sheath). Because the Ether of this state no longer conceives of itself as individual with a name and a form, the ego has disappeared. And since the Ether within the form-vase is of the same nature of the Ether outside the vase, the next step is to recognize oneself as all-pervading Ether. Every form-vase appears and disappears and, therefore, only those who are identified with the form-vase can speak of birth and death, of transmigration, of time and space, etc.

After all it is the universal Consciousness (*Īśvara*-Being) that takes different forms and particularizes («with a "part" of Myself I manifest myself»[1]), and the identification of the Ether within the vase with the different forms causes the birth of a separate individuality. In addition this is the means whereby the wheel of becoming moves. As long as there is identification there also are the I and the you, manifestation, objectification and a seeing of oneself as other than oneself.

When the Ether within the vase recognizes itself, factually and not theoretically, for what it really is, it "comprehends" the vase, with all of its different qualifications, it transcends it. It then integrates *Īśvara*-Being, as the prime cause of its exteriorization, and it resolves itself into the One-without-a-second or *nirguṇa*.

28. The *jiva* within the vase is a moment in consciousness of *Īśvara*, which corresponds to the principle-universal *Jīva* who, in turn, is a moment in consciousness of *Brahman nirguṇa* or of the non-qualified and metaphysical Being.

The bodies-vases are fed by the Ether-*Īśvara*, i.e. by the prime cause or by the seed-principle (corresponding to the microcosmic "Am"). According to Plato, all of nature, including our bodies-vehicles, is objectified and activated by the "World of Ideas". This seed has the power to move from potency to act with extraordinary, albeit relative force, and is therefore subject to being transcended. This allows us to deduce that the ego, as a separating factor, does not exist. It is pure illusion. We are not, nor could we ever be, separated

---

[1] *Bhagavadgītā*, X, 42. (Quotation marks added).

from the Ether-Being. If we believe that we are separated, this is only apparent, it is utopian. The consequence is that there is nothing to be conquered, nowhere to go, nor faraway goals to reach. There is only to awaken to the awareness of *being that which is*.

29. The Reality without a second that you are was never born, nor can it ever die, it has always been and always will be. Reality needs not realize itself, who does is its *reflection*, which lives through the contingencies of time and of effects. Reality is beyond the states of waking, dreaming and deep dreamless sleep. The whole universe, with all of its indefinite, albeit aleatory, possibilities of expression, rotates around a constant Center which does not depend on any chance or circumstance, while these depend on That.

Until you have not discovered yourself as such Reality, you may believe yourself to be many beautiful things and, although multiplicity, you will find yourself in a state of illusion. You will, therefore, remain a prisoner of those "appearances" which time offers you in order to stun you and make you forget the restless state you are in.

30. If you asked the empirical ego whether you can realize what we have said so far, it will answer that it is impossible.

This is to prove that it is not appropriate to disturb those who are completely fused with their ego-product and therefore with their sheaths-vases.

But if you start "observing" or, better still, being aware of the movement of your psyche: i.e. thoughts, emotions, desires, instincts, etc., which belong to the bodies-vehicles, you will notice that although difficult, it is not impossible. It is a question of *patience, perseverance* and thirst for completeness and freedom from the identifications with what we are not.

As we have already said and notwithstanding life's circumstances, which are always contingent even if at times quite painful, you should go on *separating* the Presence-ether that is aware of the observed. You will realize, as you certainly had the chance of noticing before, that within you everything comes and goes, everything appears and then disappears, to the exception of that conscious Presence, which never disappears. In fact, It is aware of the absence or presence of any movement that might occur within your circumference.

We are so used to "feeling alive", and that just when we are expressing our thoughts, feelings and so on, that we have no idea of a state of Being without duality. Nor can we conceptualize that condition, as it would be to no avail. This Presence is a state to be realized beyond any mental motion, because it is behind the mind, and the mind is just a simple means of expression, a body-vase.

This is why we often speak to you of realization, of attention in consciousness, etc. A person who is completely fused with his mind tool wants at all costs to understand what cannot be understood by means of mere conceptualization. The question here is not so much to understand but *to be*, and nothing else; and what is needed in order *to be* is just to realize total *consciousness*. It is only when the vehicles, which are instruments of rapport and relation, are silent that you can *discover yourself* and be what you really are; and this state will offer you fullness and therefore freedom and bliss. You can then offer this fullness to anyone, out of a pure act of love-donation and, at last, without any expectation, projection, desire or appropriation.

GLOSSARY

Advaita (n): non-duality. Absence of duality.

Ahaṁkāra (m): "what makes up the ego", sense of the empirical ego.

Apara-vidyā (f): non-supreme knowledge.

Ātman (n): the Self, the Spirit, the pure Consciousness, the ontological I.

Āvaraṇa śakti (f): the veiling power.

Avidyā (f): non-knowledge, ignorance of one's own essence.

Brahman (m) or *Brahma* (n): the absolute Reality. *Nirguṇa* (non-qualified), *Saguṇa* (qualified).

Cakra (n): "wheel", "center". The *cakras* represent determinations of the energy-awareness or *śakti*.

Chóra (χώρα): space, form in which a thing is found, common ground in which various forms follow each other, essence of matter.

Darśana (n): "point of view" on the *Veda* doctrine, philosophical school. The six main schools are: *Sāṁkhya*, *Yoga*, *Vaiśeṣ ika*, *Nyāya*, *Pūrva Mīmāṁsā* and *Vedānta*.

Diánoia (διάνοια): empirical discoursive mind, mental process, opinion.

Ens (n) lat. (pl. *entia*): being with all of its manifest vehicles, integral being. Also, impersonal individuality, universal being, divine Person, supreme Being.

Entia: see *Ens*.

Īśvara (m): "divine Person", personified God, the first determination of the absolute *Brahman*.

Jiva (m): living being. Individuated Soul. Reflection of the *ātman* on the universal plane.

Jīvanmukta (pp): "liberated during life". He who has extinguished the threefold Fire.

Manas (n): formal imaginative mind. Individuated empirical mind endowed of rational-analitical ability.

Mantra (m): sacred word or formula. Power words or sounds.

Māyā (f): phenomenon, the world of names and forms as vital phenomenon. Sensible world.

Mens informalis: higer intellect, non formal supraindividual mind.

Nóesis (νόησις): intellection, super-conscious intuition, pure intellect, intelligible knowledge.

Noûs (νοῦς): supreme intelligence, pure intellect, supreme Spirit.

Paravidyā (f): ultimate, supreme knowledge.

Prakṛti (f): nature, universal substance, *natura naturans*, the substance by which all sensible and intelligible forms are made.

Puruṣa (m): Being, man, person, the Self, the Spirit.

Sādhanā (f): ascesis, spiritual discipline, effort undergone for realization by the disciple.

Self: Spirit, the Absolute in the individual, Essence of the Being as reflection of *Brahman*.

One-One: for Plato is the Absolute non-qualified, the One of Plotinus, it corresponds to the *Brahman nirguna* of the *Vedānta*.

One-without-a-second: *Advaita*, corresponds to Plato's One-One.

Vedānta (m): "the accomplishment of the *Vedas*". One of the six *darśanas*, also called *Uttara Mīmāṁsā*.

Vidyā (f): knowledge, knowledge of reality.

Vikṣepa śakti (m): the projecting power.

RAPHAEL

Unity of Tradition

Having attained a synthesis of Knowledge (with which eclecticism or syncretism are not to be associated), Raphael aims at "presenting" the Universal Tradition in its many Eastern and Western expressions. He has spent a substantial number of years writing and publishing books on spiritual experience and his works include commentaries on the *Qabbālāh*, Hermeticism and Alchemy. He has also commented on and compared the Orphic Tradition with the works of Plato, Parmenides and Plotinus. Furthermore, Raphael is the author of several books on the pathway of non-duality (*Advaita*), which he has translated from the original Sanskrit, offering commentaries on a number of key Vedantic texts.

With reference to Platonism, Raphael has highlighted the fact that, if we were to draw a parallel between Śaṅkara's *Advaita Vedānta* and a Traditional Western Philosophical Vision, we could refer to the Vision presented by Plato. Drawing such a parallel does not imply a search for reciprocal influences, but rather it points to something of paramount importance: a sole Truth, inherent in the doctrines and teachings of several great thinkers, who although far apart in time and space, have reached similar and in some cases even identical conclusions.

One notices how Raphael's writes from a metaphysical perspective in order to manifest and underscore the Unity of Tradition, under the metaphysical perspective. This does not mean that he is in opposition to a dualistic perspective, or to the various religious faiths, or "points of view".

A true embodied metaphysical Vision cannot be opposed to anything. What is important for Raphael is the unveiling, through living and being, of that level of Truth which one has been able to contemplate.

Writing in the light of the Unity of Tradition Raphael's works present, calling on the reader's intuition, precise points of correspondence between Eastern and Western Teachings. These points of reference are useful for those who want to approach a comparative doctrinal study and to enter the spirit of the Unity of Teaching.

For those who follow either an Eastern or a Western traditional line these correspondences help us comprehend how the *Philosophia Perennis* (Universal Tradition), which has no history and has not been formulated by human minds as such, «comprehends universal truths that do not belong to any people or any age». It is only for lack of "comprehension" or of "synthetic vision" that one particular Branch is considered the only reliable one. Such a position can but lead to opposition and fanaticism. What can degenerate the Doctrine is either a sentimental, fanatical devotion or condescending intellectualism, which is critical and sterile, dogmatic and separative.

In Raphael's words: «For those of us who aim at Realization, our task is to get to the essence of every Doctrine, because we know that just as Truth is one, so Tradition is one even if, just like Truth, Tradition may be viewed from a plurality of apparently different points of view. We must abandon all disquisitions concerning the phenomenal process of becoming, and move onto the plane of Being. In other words: we must have a Philosophy of Being as the foundation of our search and of our realization»[1].

Raphael interprets spiritual practice as a "Path of Fire". Here is what he writes: «...The "Path of Fire" is the pathway each disciple follows in all branches of Tradition; it is the Way of Return. Therefore, it is not the particular teaching of an individual nor a path parallel to the one and only Main Road... After all, every

---

[1] See, Raphael, *Tat tvam asi*, That thou art, Aureā Vidyā, New York.

disciple follows his own "Path of Fire", no matter which Branch of Tradition he belongs to».

In Raphael's view, what is important is to express through living and being the truth that one has been able to contemplate. Thus, for each being, one's expression of thought and action must be coherent and in agreement with one's own specific *dharma*.

After more than thirty-five years of teaching, both oral and written, Raphael is now dedicating himself only to those people who wish to be "doers" rather than "sayers", according to St. Paul's expression.

Raphael is connected with the *maṭha* founded by *Śrī Ādi* Śaṅkara at Śṛṅgeri and Kāñcipuram as well as with the Rāmaṇa Āśram at Tiruvannamalai.

Founder of the Āśram Vidyā Order, he now dedicates himself entirely to spiritual practice. He lives in a hermitage connected to the *āśram* and devotes himself completely to a vow of silence.

* * *

May the Raphael Consciousness, expression of Unity of Tradition, guide and illumine along this Opus all those who donate their *mens informalis* (non-formal mind) to the attainment of the highest known Realization.

PUBLICATIONS

Books by Raphael
published in English

At the Source of Life
Aurea Vidyā, New York

Beyond the illusion of the ego
Aurea Vidyā, New York

Essence and Purpose of Yoga
The Initiatory Pathways to the Transcendent
Element Books, Shaftesbury, U.K.

Initiation into the Philosophy of Plato
Aurea Vidyā, New York

Orphism and the Initiatory Tradition
Aurea Vidyā, New York

Pathway of Fire, Initiation to the Kabbalah
S. Weiser, York Beach, Maine, U.S.A.

The Pathway of Non-duality, Advaitavāda
Motilal Banarsidass, New Delhi

Tat tvam asi, That thou art,
The Path of Fire According to the Asparśavāda
Aurea Vidyā, New York

The Threefold Pathway of Fire
Aurea Vidyā, New York

Traditional Classics
in English

Śaṅkara, *Ātmabodha**, Self-knowledge. Aurea Vidyā , New York

Śaṅkara, **Drigdriśyaviveka***, Discernment between *ātman* and non-*ātman*. Aurea Vidyā, New York

Gauḍapāda, **Māṇḍūkyakārikā***, The Māṇḍūkya Upaniṣad with the verses-*kārikā* of Gauḍapāda and Commentary by Raphael. Aurea Vidyā, New York

Parmenides, **On the Order of Nature**, Περί φύσεως**, For a Philosophical Ascesis. Aurea Vidyā, New York

Śaṅkara, **Vivekacūḍāmaṇi***, The Crest-jewel of Discernment. Aurea Vidyā, New York

Forthcoming Publications
in English

Patañjali, **The Regal Way to Realization***, Yogadarśana

Śaṅkara, **Aparokṣānubhūti***, Self-realization

Raphael, **The Science of Love**

The Bhagavadgītā*

Bādarāyaṇa, **Brahmasūtra***

Five Upaniṣads*, Īśa, Kaivalya, Sarvasāra, Amṛtabindu, Atharvaśira

* Translated from the Sanskrit, and Commented, by Raphael
** Edited by Raphael

Aurea Vidyā is the Publishing House of the Parmenides Traditional Philosophy Foundation, a Not-for-Profit Organization whose purpose is to make Perennial Philosophy accessible.

The Foundation goes about its purpose in a number of ways: by publishing and distributing Traditional Philosophy texts with Aurea Vidyā, by offering individual and group encounters and by providing a Reading Room and daily Meditations at its Center.

* * *

Those readers who have an interest in Traditional Philosophy are welcome to contact the Foundation at the address shown on the colophon page.